Guiding Light: Compassionate Conversations with a Parent Facing Alzheimer's and Dementia

Evelyn K. Grace

Introduction

In the delicate journey of caring for a parent with Alzheimer's or dementia, finding meaningful ways to connect becomes an essential thread in the tapestry of love and understanding. "Guiding Light" is a heartfelt guide, offering a collection of compassionate conversation ideas designed to foster connection and nurture the bond between you and your loved one.

Alzheimer's and dementia can alter the landscape of memories, sometimes leaving us searching for common ground. This short book recognizes the challenges families face and aims to be a gentle companion, providing realistic yet compassionate strategies for engaging in conversations that honor the essence of your parent's being.

As we embark on this journey together, let's navigate the intricacies of communication with sensitivity and love. Each conversation idea within these pages is crafted to spark connection, inviting your parent into a world where memories, though fragile, can still bloom. Remember, in every shared moment, you become a guiding light, illuminating the path of connection even in the midst of memory's shadows.

May these discussions serve as bridges between the past and present, offering solace, understanding, and a reminder that, despite the challenges, the love you share is a resilient force.

30 Discussions Ideas

Engaging in conversations with a parent who has Alzheimer's or dementia requires patience, empathy, and understanding. Here are 30 discussion ideas that can be adapted based on your parent's interests, memories, and cognitive abilities:

- **Family Stories:**
Share and reminisce about family stories and events from the past. Focus on positive and familiar memories.

- **Favorite Hobbies:**
Discuss their favorite hobbies or activities. It could be gardening, cooking, painting, or any other pastime they enjoyed.

- **Music Memories:**
Play music from their era and talk about the memories associated with certain songs or musicians.

- **Photo Albums:**
Look through photo albums together, prompting discussions about people, places, and events.

- **Daily Routines:**
Discuss their daily routines and reminisce about specific routines or habits they used to have.

- **Travel Memories:**
Talk about places they have visited or would like to visit. Share travel experiences and ask for their favorite destinations.

- **Favorite Foods:**
Discuss favorite foods and recipes. Share cooking memories and maybe even cook together if feasible.

- **Nature and Outdoors:**
Talk about nature, plants, or outdoor activities. Consider looking at nature pictures or taking a short walk if possible.

- **Art Appreciation:**
Discuss art, whether it's paintings, sculptures, or other forms. Visit an art museum or appreciate art at home.

- **Pets:**
If they had or have pets, discuss fond memories of them. Consider bringing in a friendly pet for interaction.

- **Favorite Books/Movies:**
Talk about their favorite books or movies. Share quotes or scenes from beloved stories.

- **Historical Events:**
Discuss historical events from their lifetime. Encourage them to share their experiences and perspectives.

- **Mindfulness and Relaxation:**
Practice simple mindfulness or relaxation exercises together, focusing on the present moment.

- **Spirituality:**
Discuss spiritual beliefs or memories of religious or meaningful events.

- **Technology Nostalgia:**
Talk about technological changes over the years. Discuss their experiences with older technology.

- **Weather Talk:**
Discuss the weather or seasons, linking them to specific memories or activities associated with different times of the year.

- **Jokes and Humor:**
Share light-hearted jokes or funny stories. Laughter can be a great way to connect.

- **Name That Tune:**
Play a "name that tune" game with music from their era. This can stimulate memory recall.

- **Gardening Conversations:**
If they enjoyed gardening, discuss plants, flowers, or gardening tips. Consider having a small indoor plant.

- **Sensory Activities:**
Engage in sensory activities, like touching different textures or smelling familiar scents.

- **Coloring or Art:**
Engage in simple coloring or art activities. This can be both relaxing and stimulating.

- **Word Games:**
Play word games or simple crossword puzzles. This can help maintain cognitive function.

- **Famous Quotes:**
Share and discuss famous quotes. Ask for their interpretations or memories related to certain quotes.

- **Fashion Memories:**
Discuss fashion trends and memorable outfits they used to wear. Look through old fashion magazines together.

- **Sports Memories:**
Talk about favorite sports teams, games, or personal experiences with sports.

- **Occupational Memories:**
Discuss their past occupations and work experiences. Share stories from their professional life.

- **Crafts and DIY:**
Engage in simple crafts or DIY activities. This can provide a sense of accomplishment.

- **Dreams and Aspirations:**
Discuss their dreams and aspirations. Encourage them to share stories about what they wanted to achieve in life.

- **Tea or Coffee Time:** Enjoy a cup of tea or coffee together. This can be a relaxing and comforting activity.

- **Reflect on the Present:** Discuss and appreciate the current moment. Share positive affirmations and express love and gratitude.

Remember to be flexible and patient, adjusting the topics based on their responses and comfort level. Always prioritize creating a positive and supportive environment for your parent.

www.ingramcontent.com/pod-product-compliance
Lightning Source LLC
Chambersburg PA
CBHW060851260726
48661CB00002B/735